Meditation For Beginners

The Guide On How To Relax, Destress And Gain Inner Peace With Your Mind And Soul

Renae K. Elsworth

Table of Contents

Bluesource And Friends

Introduction

Chapter 1: What Is Meditation?

Chapter 2: The Benefits of Meditation

Chapter 3: Observing Your Mind

Chapter 4: Getting Started

Chapter 5: Breathing Meditation

   The Stimulating Breath (or the Bellows Breath)

   The 4-7-8 (or the Relaxing Breath)

Chapter 6: Body Scan Meditation

Chapter 7: Visualization in Meditation

Chapter 8: Meditation on the Move

   The Short Path

   Tich Nhat Hanh's Walking Meditation

Chapter 9: Achieving Mindfulness in All Parts of Life

Chapter 10: Loving-Kindness Meditation

Conclusion

Bluesource And Friends

This book is brought to you by Bluesource And Friends, a happy book publishing company.

Our motto is **"Happiness Within Pages"**

We promise to deliver amazing value to readers with our books.

We also appreciate honest book reviews from our readers.

Connect with us on our Facebook page www.facebook.com/bluesourceandfriends and stay tuned to our latest book promotions and free giveaways.

Don't forget to claim your FREE books!

Brain Teasers:

https://tinyurl.com/karenbrainteasers

Harry Potter Trivia:

https://tinyurl.com/wizardworldtrivia

Sherlock Puzzle Book (Volume 2)

https://tinyurl.com/Sherlockpuzzlebook2

Also check out our best seller book

https://tinyurl.com/lateralthinkingpuzzles

Introduction

Congratulations on getting *Meditation for Beginners: The Guide on How to Relax, Destress, and Gain Inner Peace with Your Mind and Soul* and thank you for doing so.

The following chapters will discuss everything you need to know to get started with meditation practice in your life. We will discuss basic meditation skills, the benefits of meditation, habits you can use to meditate regularly, and several specific types of meditation. There is nothing necessarily religious about it and we will approach the topic from a point of view that anyone can understand. The benefits of meditation are something that all humans, regardless of beliefs, can access. Meditation is not complicated, and anyone can learn how to do it. All you need to do is have the courage to get started. Downloading this book is the first step to a life-long journey.

Beginning meditation is one of the best choices you can make to improve your life in every way. Everybody struggles and goes through difficult things but centering your mind and finding peace in meditation can help you endure. I write this book without knowing the details of your life, but I do know that you will be able to flourish. This book will help you along that process with kindness and a little bit of a sense of humor.

There are plenty of books on this subject on the market, so thanks again for choosing this one! Every effort was made to ensure it is full of as much useful information as possible; please enjoy!

Description

Your life is busy and stressful. You have a lot of demands on your time. Have you ever felt like you wanted to learn to just truly *relax*? Meditation can help. People who meditate have better relationships with their partners and children. You can be more productive and happier. It seems almost too good to be true, but it isn't. Countless people across millennia have meditated and gained inner peace through the contemplation of their own mind. Extensive research has shown many health and life benefits from meditation. Meditation is the perfect combination of ancient wisdom and modern science.

This book is informed by many years of study in several traditions of meditation. There is no dogma here, only time-tested tips about how to actually help you make progress. There are strategies and techniques from all around the world and every time period. Everything you need to know to get started is just inside.

Every long journey begins with an initial decision to start, and this book will help you along your path. Learn to focus and observe your own thoughts without judgment by exploring many different types of meditation. Learn how to integrate meditation in your daily life and find opportunities to practice mindfulness. Meditation is easy to learn but can only be mastered through regular and committed practice. The first step is in your hands.

Inside you will find:

- The many benefits of meditating, informed by science and the most cutting-edge research.

- Tips on how to maintain focus and gain more self-knowledge. Nobody is too easily distracted or bored to learn how to excel at mediation.

- Strategies for relaxation and concentration in every activity. Meditation is not just for yoga anymore.

- Walking meditations for when you want to explore the great outdoors.

- Body scan meditations for getting comfortable with yourself and learning about your own body.

- Visualizations to come to grips with your demons and bring yourself peace.

- Tools to develop compassion for everyone from your worst enemies to yourself.

Chapter 1: What Is Meditation?

Meditation is the art of learning how to focus—simple as that. The world is busy and complicated. Most people never slow down and focus on the simple inner workings of their own minds. There is always something to think about—work, family, money troubles, health problems. If you aren't careful, you will never let yourself simply be yourself. John Main, a meditation expert, says that, "In meditation, you are learning to be. Just to be, as you are."

We aren't used to just being ourselves. In modern life, there are so many demands on our time. We have to be parents, workers, students, children. We have to pay our taxes and the electric bill. We try to be fashionable and fit in. We try to project certain images of ourselves. We spend a lot of time thinking about what other people see when they look at us.

Meditation helps shut that incessant hamster wheel of expectations down.

Meditation helps you find peace and restful waking. It is a practice of renewal and regeneration. You will learn to let life flow within you and gain a new understanding of your place in it. All different types of meditation are focused on learning to be open to the present moment.

People often think about meditation as "emptying the mind" and there is a sense in which that is accurate. The goal is to remove the distraction. But this does not make the mind empty—what replaces all the petty demands of life is the ability to discern the rhythms of the universe and your own body. You will learn to exist within the subtle movements of your own breath.

You can think of the mind as a little pond. The world is constantly throwing stones and the wind is making waves. Little animals pop in and out. The surface is always troubled. These disturbances prevent us from seeing the exact character of the pond. Meditation helps us smooth out the disturbances and allow us to see the clarity of the water. In learning to quiet the world, you learn who you are.

Meditation is an ancient practice. *Meditate* derives from the Latin word *meditor*, which means to contemplate, and that itself comes from the Proto-Indo-European root **med-*, meaning to measure, give advice, or heal. Meditation heals and has been used to remedy pain and suffering for thousands of years. We are able to find guidance and discover new routes for our life through a close analysis of the self.

Traditions of meditation exist in every religion and spiritual practice. Most people, when they think of meditation, associate it with Eastern spiritual practices such a Buddhism. But meditation is a process of reflection similar to Christian contemplation and prayer or the Islamic repetition of the names of God. When religious people repeat a prayer that has been spoken for centuries, they are developing the ability to suspend focus on the here-and-now in the same way as meditation. People around the world and throughout the centuries have found meditation to be a way to develop the capacity for focused attention and concentration.

The Christian contemplative tradition focused on reflecting on God and opening up the mind. St. Gregory the Great described contemplation as "resting in God." This rest is not sleep or the cessation of all activity. This "rest" is about being open to the universe and to the divine. This often involves the repetition of scripture or ritualized prayers. The goal is to use familiar words as a way to open the self up to new experiences of grace.

Ancient Greek and Roman writers also described spiritual exercises involving attention. Philo of

Alexandria, a gnostic writer dating from circa 20 BCE, wrote about the importance of attention (*prosoche*) on the present moment. This attention brings our mind to the moment we are in and lets go of the past and future. We only have the capacity to act in the present, but we frequently are so focused on other times that we forget to be attentive to the now. The goal is tranquility, or *ataraxia* in Greek. *Ataraxia* is a state of being at peace, and the attentive student will be able to have peace of mind in any situation.

The word in English is often used as a translation of the Sanskrit word *dhyana*, which means trance or absorption. This word describes a state of deep concentration and focus, 0btained by contemplation on a single object and sustained by lucid awareness. It is not sleep, but it is a similar sense of peace and suspends most higher levels of mental activity. If you have done yoga, you might have heard of this concept. The *Bhagavad Gita* speaks of *Dhyana* as one of the four paths necessary to reach the summit of spirituality.

This book uses the tradition of meditation and mindfulness that first developed in the West during the 1960s. It is highly influenced by Hindu meditative techniques, but it has also found a home in the most cutting-edge psychological research. There are hundreds and hundreds of scientific studies about the benefits of mindfulness meditation, and we have discovered that it will help your life in a thousand different ways.

Regardless of the techniques used, meditation is a skill. An old saying among meditation experts is that mindfulness is easy, but remembering to be mindful is hard. When you first start, it will be easy to obtain a state of mindfulness for moments, but you will find yourself continually falling away. Thoughts and feelings will rise to the surface and interrupt your concentration. You will find yourself thinking about what you have to do the next morning or what you are going to cook for dinner. The interruption does not ruin meditation, but you must get in the habit of returning to focus. This takes practice and regular repetition.

The most important thing is to not get discouraged. You will get better every time you practice. We will talk about many ways you can integrate meditation in your everyday life and soon you will find that you don't know what you would do without it.

As you read through this book, remember that meditation works even as it isn't working. If you are trying to meditate or focus on the breath and find that your mind is distracted by other thoughts, that is meditation working, too. You learn something through what distracts you and draws your attention.

The important thing is a consistent, sincere effort. Put your heart into meditation and it will reward you.

Chapter 2: The Benefits of Meditation

If so many people over so long have practiced meditation, it must be pretty great. If you ask anyone who regularly practices meditation, they will tell you that it improves their life. Meditation is a miracle tool in the quest for happiness because it helps in every single way. Meditation will help you be more productive at work, it will help you in your marriage. It will even help your heart and gut. People who meditate are less biased and more accepting of new situations. Meditation makes the good times better and the bad times more bearable.

All these claims are not just anecdotal. Scientists have written countless studies examining the effects of meditation on people and they overwhelmingly show positive benefits.

Studies show that meditation strongly helps sharpen your attention. Habituation is a natural tendency to stop noticing new information in our environment. Meditation counters habituation and helps you integrate new information quicker and easier. An expert meditator will be the first person to notice a coworker's subtle new haircut or if the keys are slightly moved from where you thought you left them. This is actually a change in the brain—scientists have observed changes in the brain of expert meditators.

If you struggle with attention-deficit disorders, meditation might help you in particular. Scientists have found that adults with ADHD experienced a significant reduction in symptoms after training in mindfulness. Increases in attentiveness have been observed even five years after the training was completed.

Meditation also helps with stress. Stress is caused by the world throwing obstacles in your path and meditation cannot always help with that, but meditation certainly helps your body respond to problems. Long-term stress produces an inflammatory response that can cause serious damage to the body. Long term meditators showed considerably less inflammation than a control group of healthy adults. Meditation helps dampen over-active activity in our brains and allows us to be more resilient in the face of stress. The amygdala is a part of the brain that reacts to stressors by coordinating how the body is going to respond. In studies, the amygdales of people who meditate actually have more connections to the rest of the brain.

Being more resilient to stress has huge effects on your health. High stress is heavily associated with heart problems and chronic inflammation. If you have frequent stomach upsets or high blood pressure, meditation could help.

There is also some evidence that meditation can actually increase your life span! Meditators show increased activity of the enzyme telomerase, which is an enzyme that increases the life span of cells. If your cells live longer, you will live longer too.

In addition to your physical health, meditation can help your mental health. Meditation has been found to reduce anxiety and depression, increase positive mood, and decrease substance use and other self-harming activities. Especially when combined with other treatments like exercise, therapy, and prescription drugs, meditation can help someone overcome their mental illness struggles.

Meditation will also help you be more compassionate. Practicing meditation, especially loving-kindness meditation (Chapter Ten!) increases people's willingness to take action to relieve suffering. Expert meditators seem to actually feel more love than other people and their brains are built to experience good feelings more easily. A habit of meditation will help you develop into the parent or partner you want to be.

In a study looking at conflict in relationships, people who were more mindful were better able to keep their cool and returned to normal more quickly. The cortisol, a stress hormone, in the brains of meditators decreased more quickly than it did in the brains of less mindful people.

Mindfulness and meditation have also been shown to make people better parents. Mindful parenting leads to more positive behaviors in children and reduces the stress of parents of preschoolers and children with disabilities. Mindfulness activates the parts of the brain associated with empathy and emotional regulation, and parents who practice meditation had a better parent-child relationship than those who did not.

Even in sad situations where relationships are ending, meditation has been shown to help. Divorce tends to lead to a great deal of shame and self-criticism—meditation can help you learn to be more compassionate with yourself and therefore feel a little better when contemplating the changes in your life. Meditation leads to fewer intrusive, negative thoughts, fewer bad dreams, and less time spent thinking about negative things.

In general, meditation reduces focus on the negative things in life. In many ways, evolution has guided humans to focus on bad things happening to us. In the jungle, the memory of a tiger leaping out of a bush is more important to remember than the sight of a beautiful flower. In modern times, however, our brain is far too active about thinking about the negative. Our memory of negative things causes pain, stress, and bad health.

Focusing on meditation helps retrain your brain to focus on the positive. Some scientists performed a study where they showed pictures of things that evoked positive emotion (like photos of babies), and other pictures that had a negative association (like photos of people experiencing pain), to a group of people with a range of experiences with meditation. People who were more mindful had higher positive reactions to the positive photos and less negative reactions to the negative photos. It is amazing that meditation changes the very structure of your brain in a way that is perfect for making you feel happier. One overall way of thinking about what meditation does, is that it provides healthy distance to your own thoughts and the world. People often say that this-or-that "made" them feel a particular way. "Someone cut me off in traffic and that made me angry." What meditation does is reveal that this is false by providing distance between the event and the reaction. Something happens and as humans, we react. But if we develop a practice in observing and noticing those reactions, we will better develop the ability to change our responses.

Chapter 3: Observing Your Mind

Let's start meditating, right now. What are you thinking? What are you feeling? As we go about our days, we have millions of different thoughts and experiences. Most of them pass without us even noticing them. Right now, put down your Kindle or phone or whatever you are reading this on and try to figure out what you are thinking. Take twenty seconds, close your eyes, and observe your thoughts.

Are you back? I bet that was harder than it felt like it should be. We aren't used to looking at our thoughts and feelings from a remove. We normally just think things or feel things. It is a very different type of habit to notice, from a remove, what we are thinking.

That is all meditation is, learning how to notice one's own thoughts. People normally think of meditation as not thinking anything at all or removing all feelings.

They imagine a mental game of whack-a-mole, where you have a big cartoon hammer squashing every new thought as it arises.

People think that they cannot meditate because they cannot stop their thoughts, but the secret is that nobody can. Meditation is not about stopping thinking, because that is impossible.

One way to think what meditation is about, is to imagine sitting at the side of a road. Cars go by-and-by, but you are sitting there peacefully watching. Those cars are your thoughts and feelings.

Most of the time, we are anxious and unsettled, so we are not able to allow the cars past without stress. Instead of watching the cars, we run out into the road to try and stop traffic. We don't like that one car, we want it to go away, so we try to interrupt it.

Or, we get really hung up on one car in particular. We reach out and grab onto the bumper, try to hold on to it and keep it with us. This means that we are going to get dragged along behind.

This running around is restless and anxiety producing. It feeds on itself. The more anxious we get, the more likely we are to try to hold onto thoughts or willfully force them out of our minds.

Training our mind to meditate involves abandoning the effort to control our thoughts. Instead of control, we must learn to sit back and observe. It is normal to occasionally get caught up in it all and start chasing cars. Once you notice yourself focusing on a particular thought, take a breath and let it go. Return to the side of the road and just watch things pass by.

One technique that is helpful when learning to observe your thoughts is called *mental noting*. When something enters your mind, noting has you label it with a one-word description of what the intruder is. If you think something, you should label it "thinking." If you feel something, "feeling." Hear something? Label it "hearing." You should not be analyzing or judging the feeling. You are simply taking note of it.

Imagine the intrusion as a soap bubble in your mind. You note it by gently touching it with a label, popping it softly and painlessly. The touch of a label is supposed to help the intrusion fade away.

You can label with various levels of specificity. Sensations can be specified as "warmth," "cold," or "pain." Feelings can be labeled "worry," "fear," or "excitement." You can specify thinking into "planning" or "wanting."

Noting has many functions. The primary function is to anchor the meditator to the present. It forces the mind into a consciousness of itself. If you keep yourself attentive to noting every wandering thought, you will have the ability to be a quiet observer much more easily.

The second function is to help train the mind to recognize itself. One primary function of meditation is to help increase your ability to notice or understand your own mind. Forcing yourself to put a label on every thought helps you recognize the thought for what it is. Imagine that you feel a tightness in your chest. First, you can note it as "tightness." And then, once your attention is focused, you can specify "worry." The practice of noting helps you recognize yourself.

Third, it can help to establish patterns. If you find yourself saying "worry" over and over, it can help you understand where you are currently, mentally. It can also help gain distance from those patterns. The act of labeling has us "step away" and create distance from our own experiences. Sometimes strong emotion or obsessive thoughts can be overwhelming.

Noting will help you contextualize and cope with those feelings.

As you note your thoughts, keep an eye out for the "tone" of your mental voice. You should always be calm, gentle, and compassionate with yourself. Don't get impatient. Don't ever be harsh with yourself. With every new thought that crosses your mind, take a moment to relax and re-center on the label.

If you find yourself distracted by concerns about getting the right label, allow yourself to be vague. Sometimes people will even just note sensations with "here" or "this." If the noting keeps you present and calm, it has served its function.

Noting reflects an important theme in learning to meditate: the avoidance of judgment. The goal is to gain peace with what is, without wishing things were otherwise.

The concept of "beginner's mind" can help with this. When someone is very new at something, all experiences are fresh and uncomplicated. When you meet a new person, everything about them is alive with possibility. Cultivating beginner's mind is an attempt to retain that fresh sense of possibility and lack of judgment in all things. It is easy to become jaded and cynical about everything, including yourself. It is easy to think "I'm not the sort of person who can do this," or "this is not the type of situation I can solve." To act as if you did not know. To act uncertain, like the world can surprise you. With people, try not to let your actions be colored by memories and preconceptions.

You should strive to greet everything, in your mind and outside it, with openness.

Chapter 4: Getting Started

Some days, meditation will be easy. You will sit down, close your eyes, and find peace effortlessly.

More often, meditation will be hard. Our lives are busy and difficult—that has an inevitable effect on our attempts to meditate. The trick is to gently encourage yourself to keep at it and keep trying. It will get easier with practice and even a little bit will help.

If you are struggling, it is important to remind yourself that meditation always works. Even on the days when you struggle to focus and cannot keep your mind away from your troubles, meditation is helping. If you are able to find peace, then you have created peace for yourself. If your attention is drawn away to emotions or thoughts, you are at least more aware of how your mind is working.

What are the steps to getting started in meditation?

Step one: Find a time

My biggest tip is to find a regular time in your routine where you will meditate every day. We all have busy lives and it is very difficult to make time for yet another thing to do. But it is exactly that business that makes meditation so important. There is an old Zen saying: "You should sit and meditate for twenty minutes every day. If you are too busy, you should sit and meditate for an hour."

If you find a time in your day that you plan to always meditate, you will be more likely to do it. Research shows that habits are best built on a regular schedule. Some people like to meditate right when they get up or just before sleep. Others might meditate on their walk to work or before they have their first meeting of the day.

As you get more established in your meditation practice, you can find countless opportunities for meditation even at irregular times. Chapter 9 is all about that. You can meditate while waiting for coffee or while going for a run; eating dinner or during the trailers of a movie.

For now though, as you are just getting started, you should find a defined time and stick to it. Twenty minutes. If you don't have another, more convenient time, I would suggest starting first thing when you wake up, before you even have a cup of coffee.

Step two: Find a place

Once you have decided when you are going to meditate, you have to decide where. When you are more practiced in meditation, you will be able to meditate no matter what the disturbances are. As you are just getting started, however, you might want to make it a little easier on yourself and find someplace quiet.

It is also important that you have a place where no one will disturb you. Constant interruptions make focusing on your thoughts more difficult.

If you are in a situation where you cannot ensure solitude, that is okay, though. Sometimes it is frustrating to be a stay-at-home parent and have constant demands on your attention. You can still practice meditation. Think of it this way: you are getting a master class in meditation because you are continually having to do the hardest part—namely, refocusing and beginning again.

Step three: Sit comfortably

We all have the mental image of the Indian yogi sitting lotus style or cross-legged on the floor. If you are comfortable in that position, you are welcome to sit like that. Most of us have not regularly sat cross-legged since we were little kids, though, and it is not very comfortable for your knees.

In that light, feel free to use a chair. Sit with your legs uncrossed and your hands gently resting on your lap or your legs. Your palms can be up or down, it does not really matter. Try to keep your back straight, but not stiff. Avoid tension.

If you would like, use a cushion on your chair. You can also use a plush armchair or the couch, but that can sometimes make it more difficult to focus.

Step four: Close your eyes and begin

There is no inherent reason you could not meditate with your eyes open, but closing them can often help center the mind.

While meditating, you can use one of the strategies that will be described in the next several chapters, or you can simply sit in peace with yourself. The previous chapter described the strategy of "noting," and that is a core part of the meditation process. Sitting quietly and spending some time with yourself is all meditation is.

It is helpful in the beginning to set a timer for ten to twenty minutes. That way, you do not have to check how much time has passed. The passage of time while meditating can be very strange, both faster and slower.

Step five: Deal with distraction

Maybe you are hungry. Maybe there is a bill coming up that you do not know how you are going to pay. Maybe someone made you angry and you can't help but project bad thoughts in their direction. All of these things and more can become a roadblock in your attempt at meditating.

The first step in dealing with these problems is to accept them. A feeling exists, and it is not worth berating yourself or getting frustrated. The attempt to get back on track can only be hindered by focusing on self-criticism. Regardless of how it feels, feelings are only feelings. They are not good or bad. This is a practice of stability and equanimity.

Next, examine the distraction. Learn where your distractions come from and what causes them. In Buddhist teachings, the word for hindrance means "covering." In order to solve hindrances, you must uncover them and determine what lies beneath. Sometimes it is something physical; sometimes it is something emotional. Sometimes you will be able to fix the problem. Sometimes you won't.

Which leads to the last step: letting go. Sometimes this can be accomplished by releasing the emotional attachment to whatever is fueling the emotion or thought. Sometimes it involves accepting a feeling and letting it exist. If you are hungry and accept it as a fact of the moment, it becomes easier to focus.

Chapter 5: Breathing Meditation

Breathing meditation is perhaps the easiest way to begin a meditation practice. Many people never need to do anything else.

All meditation involves the cultivation of focus. Breathing meditation focuses on the breath as a way of focusing the mind. Breathing is at the core of our being. It is literally the stuff of life. It also forms a natural rhythm, reflecting the rhythm of the universe. There is expansion and contraction, much like the natural cycles of day and night, growth and decay, high tide and low tide. Breathing is something that we take for granted every day, but the breathing meditation returns our attention to this important part of life.

In order to start, follow the guidelines in Chapter 4. Find a good time and place. Sit quietly and comfortably with your back straight. Close your eyes.

When your eyes are first closed, take a few minutes to just exist. Notice whatever you are experiencing. Notice your body, notice what is going on around you. There are always little noises in the environment or small movements of the air. Your goal should be to settle down and sink into the chair.

Once you are relaxed, bring your attention to your breath. Simply breathe and do not try to manipulate it in any way. Notice how the breath moves in and out of your body as you inhale and exhale. Notice the details—the feeling of air moving through your nose, the small movements of muscles adjusting. Your clothes will shift over your body as you breathe— notice that.

As you breathe, your mind will inevitably wander. That does not matter. You aren't doing anything wrong. Part of the meditation is your mind wandering. Once you notice that you are thinking about something else, bring your attention back to the breath. Do this gently and softly, like correcting a small child.

All of your experiences, thoughts, emotions, and sensations should come and go in the background. Your focus should be on the breath. Allow everything else to drift in and out of your mind, in the same smooth and effortless way the breath moves through you.

Practice mental noting as you breathe. When a thought distracts you from the breath, label the thought and allow it to drift away. Always return your attention to the breath.

There are several variations of this meditation. The simplest is to allow yourself to count the breaths. Sometimes, when it is difficult to focus without guidance, the numbers can help. Some people keep counting always upward, allowing the numbers to climb and climb. Others count to ten and then start from the beginning again.

Another variation is known as the "stillness in the breath" meditation. Start as previously described, focusing on the inhale and the exhale. Slowly start to bring your attention to the moment where inhalation shifts to exhalation and exhalation to inhalation. There is a gap, a type of "still point." It is important to recognize that it has no substance or presence. It only exists in the absence of breath. Nonetheless, you can be aware of it. It has a presence in its absence.

Continue to bring your attention to the still point between the breaths. Much like everything in meditation, when you get distracted, slowly and gently bring your attention back to the still point. As you become more practiced, you may start to experience the still point as a continuous presence. This is a cultivation of stillness in the midst of movement. There is peace in the realization that there is always something still and quiet, even when there is action or activity. Buddhist teachings say there is an enlightenment in the space between breaths.

Another technique is to time the breaths in some way. The previous types of breathing had no manipulation or control of the breath. Your goal was only to observe what your body naturally did. The following two breathing exercises are ways to change your breathing so that you can have different types of experiences.

The Stimulating Breath (or the Bellows Breath)

The goal of this breathing exercise is to raise your energy and increase alertness. You should feel invigorated, similar to having just worked out.

- Inhale and exhale rapidly through your nose. Your mouth should be closed but relaxed. The breaths you take should be very short and equal in duration. This is noisy—you should be able to hear yourself breathe.

- Inhale and exhale three times in a row. After three cycles, breathe normally. There should be a quick movement of your diaphragm during the quick breaths, resembling a bellows.

- Do not breathe quickly for more than fifteen seconds for your first try. There is a risk of hyperventilating. As you practice, you can slowly increase the time up to one minute.

You should feel the effort in this breathing exercise throughout your chest and abdomen. The next time you need an energy boost and don't have time for a nap, try this breathing exercise.

The 4-7-8 (or the Relaxing Breath)

This breathing exercise helps you relax. Sit in the normal meditating position and place your tongue just behind your front teeth. Keep it there throughout the breathing exercise. As you are breathing, make sure to be purposeful about your inhalations and exhalations. When you exhale, try to force every bit of breath out of your body. When you inhale, fill up your entire core with air.

- Breathe in through your nose for a count of four seconds.

- Hold your breath for a count of seven. Exhale entirely, making a whooshing sound through your nose. This should take a count of eight seconds.

- That is one breath. Repeat the inhalation/exhalation cycle four more times for a total of five breaths.

- Breathe normally for a minute and then repeat the five counted breaths.

This is a tranquilizing breathing exercise. You will relax your nervous system and find peace. Repeat this exercise as many times as you can. Unlike a more formal meditation session, you can do this breathing exercise whenever you want. Try it while waiting in line at a coffee shop or just before bed.

Chapter 6: Body Scan Meditation

Body scan meditations involve bringing attention back to our body. Many of us spend much of our lives ignoring our bodies. We feel pain and soreness, so we put it out of our minds. We spend our workday at a desk, entirely focused on the work of our brains instead of our bodies. Some of us even have an immense amount of insecurity wrapped up in our bodies—especially particular parts of them.

Many people, when first introduced to the idea of body scanning, react with discomfort. Given that we spend so much effort trying to ignore the details of our bodies, it is hard to imagine that focusing on each individual part, in turn, could ever be soothing or relaxing.

However, I am confident that you will find peace in body scans. The technique of body scanning is an excellent way to find inner equilibrium and tranquility. It is also a good tool to build awareness of your physical health. If you are more acquainted with your body, it will be easier to notice when things go wrong.

To fully get the most out of body scan meditations, try to block out thirty to forty minutes. If you have less time, that is okay, but this is the sort of meditation you really should dwell on. Traditionally, this meditation is conducted lying down. I would suggest lying down on the floor, with a pillow under your head for comfort. Lying in the bed has a high risk of falling asleep! If you are falling asleep even on the floor, try sitting up.

It begins like much of the rest of your meditation practice will—close your eyes and focus on your breathing. Take some time to relax and settle into the space. Observe the sounds, smells, and sensations around you.

Once you have given yourself a couple of moments, bring your attention to your body. Notice the weight of it and the pressure you are putting on the floor. Notice the way your clothes feel against your skin.

Start with your toes. Try to focus all of your attention on your toes. Feel the way that they are touching each other and the sensations of their slight movement? Are they cold? If they are within socks or shoes, do you feel the constraint?

Move the attention to the rest of your feet. And then, after you've dwelt there, slowly move your way up your body.

As you examine each part of your body in turn, focus on the sensations you experience. You might find pain or numbness. There might be tingling or buzzing. Different parts of your body will feel differently. Take note of anything strange or unusual, but do not dwell on it now. The goal is not to judge anything about your body but to simply notice. Do not try to solve any problems you have while scanning your body.

If you do not feel any sensations, you can notice that too. Neutrality is an experience like any other. The point is to be curious and open to what you are experiencing. You should thoroughly explore the sensations in a particular body part before moving on to the next. This involves an intentional movement between close attention and releasing that attention.

You will find that your thoughts wander. Your attention cannot be fully controlled. If your thoughts drift, bring them gently back to the body part you have been scanning. As you practice in meditation, you will be able to maintain focus for longer and longer periods.

After you are finished analyzing your body, take a few moments to feel your breath again. Feel how it affects every part of your body. Breathe with your feet and your ears. And then, quietly open your eyes.

There are several variations on the body scan. One would be to allow your attention to move from body part to body part randomly based on where you feel sensation. This is distinct from what was described above, where you start from your toes and end with the top of your head.

Body scans are an excellent way to try and fall asleep. While in bed, start with your feet and imagine yourself sinking into the bed. Methodically switch your muscles off, reassuring each part of you that the day is done and that you do not have to do anything else. The experience of shutting each part of yourself off can be a good way to sink into sleep.

If you would like to feel more energized, it is useful to imagine your body filling up with light and heat. You can imagine each part of your body being suffused with the warmth of the sun and carry that feeling into whatever you do next.

Practicing body scans will help bring you comfort and security in your body, which is important because it is the only one you'll ever get.

Chapter 7: Visualization in Meditation

Sixty-five percent of people learn best through visual cues, so it is unsurprising that visualization exercises can be helpful for many people in their journey through meditation. There are many types of visualization techniques for many different purposes.

One of the most famous visualization techniques is known as *ideokinesis* or imaginary movement visualization. Pioneered by the Soviet Olympic Team in the 1970s, imaginary movement focuses on visualizing exactly what physical movement you are going to engage in. This is typically associated with athletics and has been shown to both increase performance and reduce anxiety about performance.

Visually running drills can actually fool our brain into constructing the mental pathways that will help with the actual physical movement. In the same way we feel genuine fear while watching a scary movie, our body does not know the difference between something imagined and something real.

Visualization is a little different than other forms of meditation. Most of what we have discussed previously has been focused on the here and now, bringing attention to the present. Visualization, on the other hand, is a type of contemplative practice where we examine our own minds. This means that it is typically best used when bracketed by sessions of concentration type meditation such as breathing meditations or body scans.

When practiced as a type of relaxation or self-soothing, it is often useful to visualize a favorite location or place. Imagine yourself at a childhood park or a beautiful beach. Walk yourself through each sensation. What are you seeing? What are you feeling?

What are you smelling? Make sure to try to make every detail as real as possible.

This focus can help relax your mind and put troublesome thoughts outside of your head.

A very different type of visualization technique focuses on those troublesome thoughts. Most of the exercises we have discussed in this book have been focused on avoiding or letting go of mental demons, but this visualization technique is the opposite.

All of us have mental demons sapping our strength. Instead of pushing those demons away, this technique involves imagining them and feeding them outside the body.

It starts by identifying a mental demon. Everyone has things in their lives that feel like they are draining energy and happiness. Imagine the feeling that you are having as the demon, not the event or incident itself.

If it is about a relationship, do not put the person in the place of the demon. Think about the demon you have chosen. Perhaps you can bring your mind to a particular incident that made this demon particularly relevant to you. While you dwell on it, scan your body and ask yourself, where is this demon held in my body? What is the shape, color, and texture of this demon? Is it hot or cold?

Intensify the sensation of the demon and personify it. Allow the sensation to move out of your body and become a being, with limbs and a face. Observe the demon. Examine its size, color, character, and emotional state. What is the look in its eyes?

Once you have fully imagined your demon, ask your demon what it wants and what it needs.

Then, switch places with the demon. Feel yourself settle in the demon's body. Imagine how the characteristics you previously observed feel from the inside. Notice how your own self looks from the eyes of the demon. Answer the following questions. As the demon:

> What I want is…
>
> What I really need is…
>
> When I get what I need, I will feel…

Once you have noted the answers to these questions, return to your own body. Observe the demon in front of you once more. Then, dissolve your body into energy. The energy should have the character of the feeling, that the demon said it would have when it gets what it needs. Notice the color of the energy.

Imagine this energy moving toward the demon and feeding it. Note how the demon consumes the energy. Give the demon energy until it is completely satisfied and notice how it changes in the process. Take your time with this step.

Once the demon is completely satisfied and happy, examine it. Note all the details of the being as you did with the demon before. Examine the color, the surface of its body, and its emotional state. Now that it is satisfied, ask the being how it will protect you. The demon was very powerful when it was a threat to you and it is still powerful as an ally.

As you look at it, imagine the being dissolving into light. Notice the color of the light and feel what it integrating into your body. You have taken the satisfied demon back into yourself and it has given lightness and luminosity to your entire body.

The demon thus consumed, take some time to return the attention to the breath and focus on the feeling that is present.

Chapter 8: Meditation on the Move

The meditations that we have previously discussed have focused on sitting quietly and still, but there are other forms of meditation. For some people, it can be easier to start with a walking meditation than a seated one. It gives the body something to do and might make it easier to clear the mind.

A formal walking meditation is done much slower than a normal walk. When you are engaged in a walking meditation, you coordinate your movements with the breath. Your eyes are open, but you are still focused on the movements of your body and the air in your lungs.

Ideally, you should practice in a secluded place. You can even walk inside if you have nowhere else to go. Stay away from highly populated walking areas, and it is very important you feel safe in your surroundings.

The goal is not to look at the scenery, so it is good if there is nothing distracting around.

Before you start the walking session, spend a minute or two focusing on the breath in a standing position. Stand with your feet hip-width apart and make sure that your weight is evenly distributed between both feet. Feel the solid ground underneath you. Close your eyes and scan your body, starting with your feet.

There are several techniques for walking meditation. Choose the one that resonates the most with you.

The Short Path

For this type of walking meditation, choose a straight path around forty feet long. If you can, try to be barefoot.

Stand upright, with your eyes cast downward. Some people keep their eyes half closed.

As you walk, your attention should be on the soles of your feet. Focus on the moments that they touch the ground and leave it again. Feel the way that your legs and feet tense as they lift away from the ground. When the foot makes contact with the path, focus your mind on the stability.

With each new step, re-focus the mind on the rhythm of your movement. When you reach the end of the path, come to a full stop. Turn around and come to a stop again. Take a breath and then continue on your walk.

Like other forms of meditation, when you feel your attention wander, bring it gently back to the breath. If you find yourself wanting to stand still or sit down to concentrate, feel free to do so.

If you find your attention wandering a great deal away from the souls of your feet, try noting the parts of the process. You can mentally think "stepping" or "left" and "right." You could try counting the steps up to ten.

Tich Nhat Hanh's Walking Meditation

Famous Buddhist monk Tich Nhat Hanh teaches a simplified form of the walking meditation. This technique focuses on affirmations as a way of soothing the mind.

- Walk slowly and comfortably.

- Bring your awareness to each step in the present moment.

- As you walk, breath in "in the here" and breath out "in the now."

- If that mantra does not resonate with you, use one that does. Any short and simple phrase will work.

- Enjoy every step you take. Imagine yourself kissing the ground with your feet and suffuse your entire body with love.

This form of meditation is less formal than the previous technique but can serve you well. Look for mantras that make you feel connected to the present moment and help you exist in peace with yourself. The goal is not to think about anything complicated. Instead, it is in the simplicity that great wisdom is found.

Chapter 9: Achieving Mindfulness in All Parts of Life

Mindfulness does not have to be something limited to specialized meditation sessions. Meditation is an important part of practicing mindfulness and you should definitely find time for a daily habit. At the same time, mindfulness should extend beyond that daily twenty minutes.

You can integrate mindfulness into any activity you do. This chapter will list a number of different examples of moments where you can practice mindfulness, but there are countless more. Do not be limited. Make it a game to live in the moment as much as possible.

When you are waiting in line in a coffee shop, take some time to observe the world around you. Notice the smells and sounds and soft movements of air against your skin. Be present at the moment. Take the time to really notice as many details as possible.

Pick up a familiar object. Examine it. What is the texture of it, how much does it weigh? Exactly how does it feel in your hand? What does it smell like? Focus your mind entirely on the object at hand.

Turn your chores into rituals. When you do a repetitive task, focus on the rhythm of the movement. Watch the slow progress of cleanliness spreading across the surface. When you are sweeping, listen to the sounds that the bristles make against the floor. Practice finding happiness in even the most mundane of activities.

Go for a walk outside. Unlike the formal walking meditations described in the last chapter, focus on the world around you. Notice how the sun feels against your skin, and see what you can smell on the wind.

Look for the tiny creatures all around in every public space. Try to see all the ways life is hiding.

Practice yoga or stretching. Simple, slow movements can really help center yourself in your own body. You do not have to attend classes or pay for a teacher, though that would be a great idea. YouTube has many videos of basic yoga exercises. If you do not want to do that, simply stretch. Feel your muscles moving under your skin.

Make an altar. Put photos or small, meaningful objects in a particular place in your house and take some time to contemplate during the beginning or end of your day. A few moments of quiet can help you feel more connected to the world.

While eating, focus on all the sensations in your body. Take the time to smell the food before eating it. Chew pieces of food extensively and feel the way the texture and taste change in your mouth. Focus on how you are feeling. This is a helpful way to get in tune with your body and avoid eating too much. When you really enjoy everything you consume, there is no need to flood your body with sugar and fat.

When you have a break during the day, instead of picking up your phone, close your eyes and focus on your breath. The phone is one of modern life's biggest enemies to mindfulness. There are so many ways it intrudes on our thoughts. We focus on what others are saying and doing instead of our own lives. Try to avoid social media in your life.

When you are angry or upset, take a moment to dwell on the emotion instead of harshly reacting. Strong emotion tends to make people act quickly and without thought. Get in the habit of becoming still when you feel a strong emotion. Take the opportunity to observe the emotion and exactly how it makes you feel. What does your body feel like? Where is the emotion coming from? Usually, taking these moments of stillness will allow you to think through any actions you otherwise might have thoughtlessly done in anger.

When your phone rings at work, allow it to ring a few times before picking it up. Take that moment to breathe and destress. Practice distancing yourself from the urgency of modern life. You will still pick up the phone, but you will just do so a couple of seconds later. It is easy to see every small moment as an emergency, and it is useful to practice the simple art of waiting.

Listen to music. Try to pick out every individual instrument. Focus on one instrument at a time and try to only hear that part of the song. Once you have fully understood that part of the song, pick another instrument. It is often useful to listen to the same song over and over again if you can, in order to really gain relaxation.

When you are reading and you come across a phrase or sentence that resonates with you, instead of highlighting and moving on, pause. Read the passage again and sit with it. Read it out loud and listen to the sound of the words in your own mouth. What does the passage mean to you? Does it bring up any images or memories for you? Once you have finished dwelling on the individual phrase, return to the larger work and notice if your relationship to it has changed.

Journal. Sit down with a notebook or some paper and write about your day. You can do so methodically, starting from the beginning of your day, or in a more unstructured fashion. Take some time to discover what you are thinking through writing it down.

When speaking with someone else, truly listen. Maintain an open and receptive stance, without any judgment. Try not to jump ahead in the other person's train of thought or predict what they are going to say. Do not have any agenda. As responses come up in your mind, gently release them and return your focus to what is being said. Be curious.

Chapter 10: Loving-Kindness Meditation

Loving-kindness meditation *(metta bhavana)* is an ancient Buddhist meditation, but it can be practiced by anyone regardless of religion. Loving-kindness is inclusive, unconditional love. It is love that is not about what one deserves. It is not restricted to friends or family—one can and should have loving-kindness toward the whole world. Indeed, it is important to have loving-kindness especially to those you do not otherwise like. Loving-kindness has no expectations and does not want anything in return.

Loving-kindness meditation is a practice of softening the heart and sending out warm and loving energy into the world. It involves breaking down barriers between you and the rest of humanity.

Like many of the other meditations that we have discussed in this book, start with some moments of quiet contemplation and concentration. Focus on your breathing, eyes closed and in a comfortable, seated position. After you have settled in, pull your attention in toward your heart. Breathe in and out while focusing on your heart, as if you are breathing from your solar plexus. Anchor your mind on that location. Draw out a feeling of love and safety from within yourself. Imagine your body filling up with sweet warmth, like melted chocolate.

Focus on someone you love. This should be someone who is easy to love with no expectation or sense of possession. They should evoke a feeling of pure, unconditional loving-kindness. This is usually a parent or mentor, someone toward whom it takes no effort to feel respect. Think of that person's face, their smile.

While dwelling on this person, repeat (internally or out loud) the following several times until you feel truly full of loving-kindness.

> May she be happy.
> May she be at peace.
> May she be free from suffering.

If you would like, you can replace these phrases with some that resonate or substitute specific, heartfelt wishes for this person.

You should also imagine love coming from them toward you. Imagine the warmth you feel when they look at you, and bask in the regard of their love. Take the time to soak it in, so that you can use it to cast back out into the world.

The next person you think of should be a friend and someone you feel a fondness for. While dwelling on them, repeat the same phrases several times.

Following that person, take the time to dwell on someone you feel neutral toward. Ideally, this should be a person you barely know and have no strong feelings for, either like or dislike. While you dwell on the thought of them and repeat the phrases, imagine their lives and what they value.

Next, focus on someone you dislike or have feelings of intense hostility toward. The more intense the dislike, the more effective the exercise. If you find yourself being distracted by ill-will, return to the first beloved person and dwell on them until you are filled with warmth and love once again.

Next, focus on humanity in general. Focus on all living beings and send warmth out into the universe. Feel loving-kindness expand out from your body and emanate toward all beings around you. If you find it difficult to feel love for people in general with no specific purpose for your feelings, imagine strangers in a variety of different scenarios. The person in the grocery store checking your groceries out, or a child in the library. The goal is to feel exactly the same way about every living being, that you feel about the most beloved benefactor who you started this exercise thinking about.

You can repeat this exercise, making yourself a conduit for a river of love, toward different categories of people. You can direct loving-kindness to animals, or only women, or only children. If you have found yourself struggling with empathy toward a particular group of people, take the opportunity to practice loving-kindness oriented toward that group.

Once you feel at peace with the world, move your attention back to the self. Repeat the exercise one last time, but direct the loving-kindness inward. Repeat phrases of kindness toward yourself. You are welcome to substitute specific wishes you have for yourself, but the best use of the exercise is to focus affection on parts of yourself you otherwise dislike or resent. Generate warm, loving feelings toward yourself.

Some people advise to begin with the self instead of the much-loved mentor, but we often struggle to love ourselves with the same compassion that we love other people. By starting with someone we are practiced in treating kindly, it is easier to practice that same empathy and goodwill toward everyone else in the process.

Loving-kindness, as a practice, should not just be limited to isolated moments of meditation. As you go through your life, try to engage with everyone you meet with love. Practice compassion and forgiveness toward all those who hurt you, including yourself. This is not only a way to treat other people better, but it will also pay great dividends in your own happiness. Negative emotions such as anger and hate take a grave psychic toll on most people. It is hard to feel happy and positive when much of your attention is negatively oriented toward others.

Developing the skill of loving-kindness will help you achieve peace in all your endeavors.

Conclusion

Thank you for making it through to the end of *Meditation for Beginners*. Let's hope it was informative and able to provide you with all of the tools you need to achieve your goals, whatever they may be.

The next step is to use your meditation skills in every way you can. Develop a daily practice of meditation. The first thing when you wake up, sit up in a chair, close your eyes, and focus on the breath. Develop the skills of focusing the mind and live in the present moment. Also, take that mindfulness into every part of your life. I would suggest going back to Chapter 9 on a number of occasions, and reminding yourself of all the different ways you can be mindful.

The world is busy and difficult. It is easy to forget to be mindful and at peace with yourself. The more you practice the skill, however, the easier it becomes.

Even the greatest spiritual leaders started off as novices, struggling to keep focus and keep their mind at ease. When you struggle, remember that this is only the beginning of a life-long journey.

Luckily, there are so many resources available to you that can help you on your journey. There are a variety of apps with audio meditations, if you find it easier to meditate with someone speaking. If you would not like to pay additional money for meditations, I would suggest recording yourself speaking parts of the meditations available in this book. Then, you will be able to guide yourself along the process of meditation.

If you are really enjoying meditation and want to learn more, I would suggest exploring the great spiritual traditions which have developed meditation practices. You do not have to have any particular religious commitment to learning from Buddhist and Hindu teachers who specialize in meditation. The skills they teach are relevant and useful regardless of what belief you have in God. The world is full of people with so much to teach. Engage in that world in peace and with mindfulness, always approaching new situations like a child would—with joy and without any baggage.

Finally, if you found this book useful in any way, a review on Amazon is always appreciated!

Renae K. Elsworth

Connect with us on our Facebook page www.facebook.com/bluesourceandfriends and stay tuned to our latest book promotions and free giveaways.

Made in the USA
Middletown, DE
30 April 2019